TIFFANY LE, MSN, FNP-C

LAND YOUR FIRST 6 FIGURE NP JOB

- ✓ *Get your foot in the door*
- ✓ *Sail through the interview*
- ✓ *And get the job*

Contents

Introduction 4
   A little bit about me… 4
   Different types of nurse practitioners 5

Chapter 1: Networking 7
   Network and build good relationships 7
   Ask for recommendation letters from those with higher or equivalent level of training 8

Chapter 2- The Art of Finding the Right Job 10
   Have a kick butt resume! I cannot stress the importance of this… 10
   Find the right "key words" to catch employers' attention 12

Chapter 3- Applying for that Perfect Job 14
   When you are actively searching for a job, if a strange number appears on your caller ID, do not pick up. 15
   Take clinical rotations or current RN jobs as an opportunity for you to show your skills and get that job offer. 15
   Find the recruiters and contact them directly 16
   It takes time for the right job to come along, especially as an NP, so be patient. 17

Chapter 4- The Interview 18
   There is no such thing as a bad Interview. Gather what you learned and do not make the same mistakes next time. 18
   Making your way to the interview. 21
   Treat each interview like an important test and prepare for it 21
   Ask questions during the interview 22

Chapter 5- Seal the Deal 24
   Gather a portfolio 24

Chapter 6- Keep Your Options Open 27

If the market for NP in your area is too competitive, is commuting an
  option?..27
  Negotiate your contract..27
Chapter 7- A Word Based Upon My Experience 29
Conclusion 30

Introduction

Most people I have encountered in my daily life want to know what it's like to be successful and how to gain that success. Sadly enough, the world is a harsh place, and no matter what we seem to try, we just can't get our feet in the door to seal our success. If this sounds like you, don't be afraid that success will never come for you. This just means that you need to try a new approach to finding your fit.

During my job search, I have looked at my personal journey and realized just how much my experiences can help others to find the right job. Before I begin, I would like to tell you a little bit about myself and why I'm writing this book. My experiences have been anything but easy, but I'm happy to have had them so that I can share them with others.

A little bit about me...

My name is Tiffany Le. I just recently became a Family Nurse Practitioner (FNP-C). In the past, I had been a registered nurse for almost 6 years before starting my new role as a nurse practitioner. I worked in emergency medicine for a year before I decided to get my nurse practitioner degree. Nursing is a demanding field that is very rewarding but can be exhausting and frustrating. I love helping people and their families, and I love my job.

However, as an RN, I felt overworked and underpaid. I often found myself mentally and physically exhausted, hungry, and even dehydrated by the end of my shifts. I started to find it hard to take care of my patients because I couldn't even take care of myself. How can I give what I do not have myself?

I saw the career of nurse practitioner as a great way for advancement while still helping my patients and delivering the best care for them. After I graduated with my FNP degree, I was super excited to start working. In a short time, I realized no one wanted to hire me. Why didn't I get the job? Why did some companies even pay NPs less than RNs? Why is the job market for nurse practitioner so competitive?

Statistics show that the number of nurse practitioners will increase by 35% from 2012 to 2024[1]. This means that finding nurse practitioner jobs will be more competitive than ever before. What will set you apart from the other fifty candidates? I went from no job offer to landing a $130,000* job offer my first year out of school. This does not include the continued medical education (CME) stipend, overtime, holiday pay, and bonuses. This can happen to you. Take the mistakes I made and learn from them in order to get your next six figure-income NP job offer.

And just in case you're wondering, my $130,000* a year comes with a commitment of only 144 hours a month! If you think that you have to work long hours to make this type of money, think again!

Different types of nurse practitioners

Before going much further into this book, I would like to point out that there are multiple types of nurse practitioners in the field. Finding a specialty that suits you is incredibly important if you hope to succeed in this career field. I want to take a brief look at the different types of nurse practitioners so that you can get a brief glance at what you have to choose from once you start your education.

My degree is a Master's of Science in Nursing (MSN), with an emphasis as a Family Nurse Practitioner (FNP). I find that the FNP specialty is the most widely sought after degree. It is a "generalist" degree which allows you to advance in many areas of the nursing profession. I have seen nurses with FNP degrees in education, management, and clinical jobs. I am an FNP practicing in the emergency department. I have also seen FNPs in orthopedics, surgery, and pain management. With the flexibility that it offers, I would recommend this degree over the overly specialized ones.

---

[1] U.S. Bureau of Labor Statistics. (15 December 2015). Retrieved from http://www.bls.gov/ooh/healthcare/nurse-anesthetists-nurse-midwives-and-nurse-practitioners.htm#tab-6

However, there are also specialty nurse practitioners such as pediatric, neonatal, women's health, adult, geriatric, psychiatric, or acute care NP. These degrees may limit the areas that you can practice. When weighing your options, a specialized field may pay a little more in the long run, but finding a job may be more difficult. Specialized degrees also allow you to see a certain group of patients that you are comfortable with and have a wealth of knowledge and experience with. If you wish to specialize, look at the field before going to school for this. It may save you some headaches once you graduate and begin to search for jobs.

Before seeking the education that you need to enter the field, think about your overall goals for your career. There is nothing more frustrating than going into a job that makes you miserable, no matter how good the money is.

Since I have been in the field, I have gotten a glimpse of what you should or should not do in order to find your ideal job quickly and start earning the income you deserve. In this book, I am going to give you some practical tips on how you can quickly find work and continue to grow your career into a rewarding life experience.

Chapter 1: Networking

So, you have just finished school and the world is at your fingertips. You are excited to get going, but you have no idea where you should begin. Think about this scenario from an outsider's point of view. You don't know employers, and employers don't know about you. How are you going to make your connections?

Trust me, sitting around and waiting for the offers to roll in doesn't work. No matter how excited you are, you are an unknown in the field right now. How can you get your name out there? My first piece of advice would be to start networking, even before you are finished with school.

In this chapter, I'm going to examine the benefits of networking in your field so that you are associated with employers before you start looking for your first job! You can even use these tips if you have already landed a job, but you want to accelerate your job growth as quickly as possible.

Network and build good relationships

Building relationships before or while you are working as a RN with co-workers, physicians, other NPs, physician assistants (PAs), and everyone around you is a great way to get your name out into the field. It is a good idea to network while you are still in school or just starting out. Talk to the lead providers at the current facility you work at and tell them that you are in school, your anticipated graduation date, and put yourself out there. Ask about potential job openings if you are interested in practicing there. It is always a good idea to work in the setting you'll likely want to work in as an NP. If you are an RN in a medical surgical unit, but you want to practice in emergency medicine, then find a job in an ER as an RN. Employers like to see NPs with some experience in the field they are applying to.

To give you an idea of how this can work out, let me use my experience as an example. I worked in the ER as an RN at a large hospital and wanted to work there after graduation as an NP. However, I was not offered the job. Why? I did not put myself out there while I was in school. I did not try to connect with the lead advanced practitioner or the hiring personnel while I was in school. I just emailed her one day and asked for a job. Off course, I did not get it. She had no clue who I was. For all she knew, I was a regular person with no experience to speak of.

There are more RNs going back to school and getting advanced degrees now than ever before. The jobs are competitive and you have to stand out. While you are working as an RN, you need to think like an NP. Impress the people you work with. Ask the questions about the disease process and do not be afraid to ask questions. Often times, when I ask other NPs, they do not know the answer to the questions either. At this point, we end up looking for the answers together. This simple act shows initiative and willingness to learn. It will make you be more respected as an RN and will help your future goal of obtaining an NP job.

Ask for recommendation letters from those with higher or equivalent level of training

Standing apart from the competition is important, especially in such a competitive career field. With this being said, finding people to recommend you will help set you apart from the competition. Impress the people you work with whether it is on the job, clinical rotations, or professors. Build good relationships with other nurse practitioners, PAs, physicians, and professors. All of these people can help land your next six figure income job. When you are getting ready to apply for jobs, ask them to write you letters of recommendation. The recommendation letters will set you apart from other candidates. A recommendation letter shows the hiring personnel that you're known in the field and have experience and rapport with others in the field.

While I was in school, one of my clinical rotations was in the emergency department. I worked really hard while I was there, and I asked the ER physician I trained with to write me a letter of recommendation. I told her my goal is to get an ER-NP job after graduation. Going a step further, I also got recommendation letters from other NPs and physicians I worked with and have had good relationships with over the years. I honestly believe the recommendation letters that I brought to the interview landed me the $130k offered. Potential employers are more likely to read the recommendation letters at the interview rather than calling the references you listed on your resume. By taking the time to obtain these letters, you are saving your prospective employer time by bringing the references with you.

Networking and building a rapport with colleagues can really help boost your chances of obtaining the job that you are hoping for. While it takes time and effort to get to know professionals and build these relationships, the benefits can help you throughout your entire career. The rapport that I built during my clinical rotations helped me to get the job that I wanted. While I didn't realize this in the beginning, knowing that references and networking are great tools for the employment process. I highly encourage you to start this process early on in your schooling. It could land you your dream job!

Chapter 2- The Art of Finding the Right Job

Once you are finished with your schooling, it is time to put the skills that you have learned to good use. This means it's time to find your first job! You may be thinking about this with fear. While your schooling was a great experience, you are not prepared for the real world. How can you find the job that you dream of? How can you make the income that you have heard about?

Getting out into the field can be initially intimidating, but once you have your feet wet, you are prepared for whatever the job search throws your way. However, getting to the point where you are confident with your abilities and job seeking skills takes a little time and practice. In this chapter, I am going to give you a few tips on how you can make your initial and future job searches much easier. Getting yourself prepared for the job search is the next step in landing your ideal job!

Have a kick butt resume! I cannot stress the importance of this...

The biggest mistake that you can make when applying for the job is not having a well put together resume. As an RN, I did not find a resume as imperative when applying for jobs compared to applying to nurse practitioner jobs because those jobs were abundant and less competitive. Once I started searching for nurse practitioner jobs, I found that the resume was incredibly necessary and I had to spend a lot of time and effort making it stand out from those of the competition.

There are many misconceptions about what a resume needs to incorporate. I was always taught that a resume should be one page, no more and no less. Wrong! The resume does not have to be limited to one page. Mine ended up being two pages and is still expanding as I build my experience. My biggest mistake when applying for jobs early on was my resume. I was so excited that I passed the national boards and was ready to work as a nurse practitioner that I started applying to jobs with a resume that was three years old. Sure, I updated it with my current title, but that was pretty much it. I did not include the skills, procedural experience, or qualifications I earned during my nurse practitioner schooling.

After six weeks of no call-backs or interviews, I reevaluated the situation and come to find out, it was my awful resume. I started to ask some nurse practitioners who received multiple jobs offers if they would allow me to see their resumes. When I pulled their resumes up, I felt so embarrassed. My resume was a joke! I thought, "No wonder why I did not get a single call!" I spent the next couple of days updating and adjusting my resume.

What is in a good resume? The resume should include your skills, any procedures that you have done, your awards, your GPA, your duties, qualifications, clinical sites, and whatever other information that will make you more marketable. For example, some of the skills and procedures that I put on my resume were but not limited to:

- GYN—Pelvic exams, manual exams, STI exams and treatment, STIs testing
- Respiratory: neb treatment, peak flow, spirometer
- Derm: I&D, wound care
- ENT: removal of foreign body from the eye, tx of corneal abrasion, cerumen dis-impaction, removal of a foreign body from the ear
- Orthopedic: fracture immobilization, splinting

These are the procedures that I have done in clinicals and felt comfortable in performing on a regular basis. Do not sell yourself short. Make a list of the procedures and skills you have done and include that in your resume. You may not have done any of these as much as you would like, but doing them to begin with gives you experience which you can build upon.

Another piece of advice that I want to give when it comes to your resume: don't inflate your skills and experiences. If you have heard about it, but you have not actually been trained to or done the procedure, don't put it on your resume. Over-qualifying yourself can be just as harmful as understating your abilities.

Find the right "key words" to catch employers' attention

Typically, large companies have a system to filtering out candidates before a resume will even reach a recruiter's hands. If your resume passes these filters, it reaches a recruiter. The recruiter of the company will then call to set up a time to talk. If they feel you are a good fit, then they will forward your resume to the hiring manager. So, what do these recruiters look for? How can your resume pass the initial filter?

Recruiters look for keywords. They want to make sure that you have read and understand the job, and your resume is a reflection of whether or not this is the case. So, when I was applying for jobs, I looked for key words in the job descriptions before submitting my resume. I made sure to adjust my resume to include the key words. For example, one job description was "provider must be able to interpret labs, make diagnoses, and perform comprehensive physical exams". Those are "key words" that should be included in your resume. During my NP training, I did all those things. Therefore, under my professional summary, I listed:

- Perform health history and physical exam
- Gather appropriate supporting data and identify problems
- Interpret and evaluate labs and diagnostic tests
- Make medical diagnosis and institute therapy or referrals appropriately
- Construct a plan of care/ action for further testing if required
- Provide instructions and guidance to patients regarding medical care
- Knowledge and experience with Electronic Medical Record
- Bilingual, speaks Vietnamese and English fluently
- Enthusiastic and fast learner
- Provides great customer service

Smaller companies and private practices typically do not have the filtering software. With that said, your resume should still include keywords from the job description for consideration with the company. This shows attention to detail and that can help put you in a better standing when they decide who to interview for the position.

The resume is important. It's an introduction to yourself even before an employer has the opportunity to meet you. You want to make a good impression from the beginning. Sure, you may have to tweak your resume for individual jobs, but having a solid resume to begin with will make this process easier and less time-consuming.

Now that you have a great resume, the next step is to put yourself out there and begin applying for your ideal job! In the next chapter, I will give you some tips on how to apply for a job and stand out amongst other applicants. Learning these skills before the job search will make the process faster and more productive!

Chapter 3- Applying for that Perfect Job

Applying for your first position in your new field can be intimidating. Since the competition is intense in this field, you may feel like you don't have a chance against more experienced applicants. The first piece of advice that I will give you is to push those thoughts aside. You have to have confidence in yourself and your abilities, or you won't get the job that you want.

Do you have an ideal job in mind? Start your search in that area. Look for the expectations that you have for the job and begin your search there. What do you see as your job duties? What kind of patients do you wish to work with? Do you have a specialty area that you can narrow down the search with?

I started searching for jobs two weeks before I took my national board exam to see the possibilities the field offered. I started applying for jobs seriously after I pass my national boards. I passed these crucial exams on May 3, 2016, a day I will never forget. Even though I waited to apply for jobs until after I was certified, you can certainly apply beforehand. I started applying for jobs I only wanted in my area, limiting my possibilities to the Emergency Department. After two weeks of no response and no interview, I began to panic. The thoughts of getting my NP degree without an NP job scared me. I also knew a few NPs who couldn't find jobs as nurse practitioners and continued to work as RNs instead. I certainly didn't want to be in that position and neither should you. Other thoughts haunted me, such as the fact that I had student loans I needed to pay for and two babies I needed to feed (a 20 month and 4 month old).

When I began my job search and had no response, I felt as though my education had been for nothing. Had I just wasted my time only to return to my job as an RN? Fortunately, this scenario did not play out as I feared. The calls began to come in soon enough, and I found myself beginning to interview for NP jobs. In this chapter, I am going to give you some hints on ways that you can be prepared for your job search and how you can make your search turn into an interview.

When you are actively searching for a job, if a strange number appears on your caller ID, do not pick up.

After a few weeks of silence from all the employers I applied to, I started applying for anything that was available, even things I have no experience with or business applying to, such as surgery. Desperation makes you do things that you probably wouldn't ordinarily do. I was surprised when one day a recruiter called me about a surgical nurse practitioner position that I had applied to. She asked why I wanted to be a surgical nurse practitioner, and the only running through my head was "I need a job." Of course, I could not tell her what I was really thinking, and I quickly scrambled for a good response and made something up.

I made a few mistakes when I answered this call. When the recruiter called, I was at the grocery store and running around. My mind was not on my job situation or talking to a recruiter about a job that I wasn't qualified for. Mentally, I was not ready to answer her questions and distracted by something completely unrelated to what she wanted to talk about. As you may have already guessed, I did not hear back from her.

The point I am trying to make is do not pick up for strange numbers during your job search. Let the phone go to your voicemail. Allow the person to leave a message. This is a good way to prepare yourself for what they might asked and the type of position it is. If you have applied for multiple positions, you will also know who is trying to reach you and you can call back with a focus for what the job is and what you need to do to prepare for a phone screening.

Take clinical rotations or current RN jobs as an opportunity for you to show your skills and get that job offer.

Your first place to begin your job search should be the place that you are currently working. Clinical rotations are a great way for you to land your first job offer. Every time I went to clinical, I viewed this as an opportunity for a potential job offer. I worked really hard while in my clinicals and built a good relationship with the staff members who worked there. I was fortunate to receive two different job offers from my clinical sites. Even though I had to choose one over the other, I would rather have multiple offers that allow me to pick than no offers and having to settle on something I don't necessarily want to do.

If you are needing to work and still haven't found the right fit for you, don't be afraid to take a few RN jobs to get in the door. This will allow you to show your other skills off and let new places know that you do have training as an NP. Even though this is below your field, you can still find opportunities to learn and grow that will help you in the future.

Find the recruiters and contact them directly

When beginning your job search, the internet is an invaluable tool to help you find opportunities near you without having to do a ton of foot work. While there are numerous sites out there that can help find you the right job, some are more helpful than others. The search engines that I found most useful were Indeed, Glassdoor, healthcare career connections, staffing agencies, and large hospitals in the area. It is a good idea to set up job alerts on these sites so you will see new job postings as they become available.

I also created a LinkedIn account. This is a social media site tailored to career-minded individuals. You can network with those in your field and get a feel for the people who you are most likely to work with. It is important to have a professional profile picture and some good facts about yourself and your qualifications. After I set up my LinkedIn account, I noticed recruiters were looking at my profile before contacting me. I also searched for recruiters through LinkedIn and tried to connect with them directly.

Another great feature of online job searches is that I could send my resume directly to the recruiters of that company I was applying to. I realized quickly that I received a better response that way. Some recruiters were helpful and forwarded my resume to the hiring manager. Other recruiters just did not respond. Even though it didn't work well in all circumstances, I still found that it was a good way to market yourself.

It takes time for the right job to come along, especially as an NP, so be patient.

If you are applying for NP jobs aggressively, it typically takes three to four months to find the right job. For over a month after applying aggressively, I still did not receive any interviews, calls, or emails from any potential employers. This was really discouraging. After I updated my resume and fixed some the mistakes I mentioned earlier, I still did not receive any calls for some time. This started to get depressing. I began to wonder what was wrong with me. I talked to other NPs and asked how long it took them to get their job. The most frequent response was about three months. They advised me to be patient because it takes time for the right job to come along. However, you do not want it to take too long.

NPs who have been out of school for too long and have not practiced will make employers see you as a "red-flag". For example, if you graduated three years ago with your NP degree and still working as an RN, potential employers may wonder why. Make sure you have a good reason for this choice of job if that is your case.

While you might be ready to start working in your new job tomorrow, it takes time for employers to find the right candidates and bring them into their practice. Remember this if you feel as though you haven't been getting the responses that you hoped for in the beginning. If you find that you're not getting responses at all, take a look at your approach and even your resume. Maybe you're not marketing yourself in a way that catches an employer's attention.

Finding and applying for jobs in your new field can be a long and stressful process. We have all been through it and have learned from it.

Take this as a learning and growing experience for the next time you are looking for a new position.

The next step is to be prepared when that offer for an interview comes!

Chapter 4- The Interview

All of us have been through the interview process before, even if it was for a fast food job. It is an exciting and scary time. However, it is something that you have been working towards and you want to be prepared for.

Finally it came: my first interview! I was so excited! It was also an emergency medicine job, which was where I really wanted to be. The hiring physician, Dr. Adam, told me to come in and shadow him. At first, I thought that would be the whole interview. I was so excited and quickly scheduled something for the next day. What a mistake! As I prepared for the shadowing, I was thinking to myself, *I got this job*. I had been an emergency room RN for almost four years at a level one trauma center, I was more than prepared for the job offer. *Job secured*, I thought. Oh, what a rude awakening.

Before I went on the interview, I asked a fellow NP how her recent job shadow went. She stated, "I was given a tour of the department and answered some basic interview questions and two weeks later I got the job." She also encouraged me by telling me that if the physician is willing to meet with you, "you pretty much already have the job, and they do not have that much time to waste." I felt at ease talking to her and was excited to meet Dr. Adam. However, my experience was nothing like that of my fellow NP.

There is no such thing as a bad interview. Gather what you learned and do not make the same mistakes next time.

I was going to meet Dr. Adam at 6am the next morning so I went to bed at 9pm the night before to make sure that I had a full night's rest. That night, my 3 month old kept waking up during the night, so I did not get any sleep. With no sleep and feeling extremely tired, I was exhausted before the day even started. To make matters worse, I was also running late that morning and did not get any breakfast.

I got there exactly at 6am and met Dr. Adam. He introduced me to the providers that were there. After I greeted some providers, he turned to me and handed me a patient's chart. Dr. Adam stated, "This patient is here for abdominal pain. I want you to go see her then come report to me what you find." I was stunned! I was not ready or mentally prepare for this. I panicked! I thought I was here so he can show me around the department, tell me about the company, and then offer me the job. I did not know I was going to be tested! Shouldn't I had been warned about this?

I had to close my eyes and take a deep breath before going in. After I interviewed the patient and perform a physical exam, I reported to Dr. Adam. I quickly ran through why the patient was there, stated some differential diagnoses, and some diagnostic tests I wanted to order on her. He interrupted and stated, "You need to gather your thoughts Tiffany and present this patient to me as a provider." My face turned hot red. I was so nervous and scared by this time. "You went from chief complaint to wanting to order labs on the patient," said Dr. Adam while shaking his head. Another physician that was sitting nearby looked at me to see my reaction and quickly looked away. I thought I was going to cry at that instant. I tried so hard not to cry and tried to remain composed.

There I was, just graduated from NP school and so proud of myself. At this moment I have no self-esteem and felt so small. Dr. Adam told me to gather my thoughts again and present this case to him in ten minutes. I nodded and got busy writing down every single word I would say. I started with the history of the present illness that included a detailed history of subjective review of systems, objective findings, differential diagnoses, evaluations, and a plan for the patient. After presenting the patient to Dr. Adam the second time, he agreed with my evaluation and plan. I exhaled and felt a brief second of relief until he tossed me another chart. I looked at my watch and realized that it was only 8am. I thought to myself, *this will be a long day.*

My next patient came in for chest pain. I was determined to do well this time because I wanted to impress Dr. Adam. I interviewed the patient, asked all the appropriate questions, and did my physical assessment. I wanted to be ready and wrote down exactly what I would say, my evaluation and plan for the patient. When I presented to Dr. Adam that the patient came in for chest pain, he immediately asked me, "Tell me seven things you want to rule out immediately if a patient is having chest pain."

My jaw dropped. He sat directly across from me and looked me right in the eye, holding seven fingers up. I scrambled to say something so I wouldn't look like a total dunce. "Well, um…myocardial infraction," I said nervously. He continued to look straight at me with six fingers still up. "Um, pulmonary embolism, pneumothorax, aortic aneurysm," I stuttered while hoping he will tell me the last three. However, he continued to look at me with 3 fingers held up. Meanwhile, it is dead silent in the room for at least a minute. I finally thought to myself, *this man will not let me off the hook.* I ended up telling him I could not name the last three. He told me, "esophageal rupture, cardiac tamponade, and sometimes pneumonia." I nodded and felt relieved that that painful question was over. But behold, he then asked, "so Tiffany, tell me how you rule out cardiac tamponade and the other six emergent situations?" I froze and wanted to give up and go home.

I do not know why but I stuck around to get tortured some more. Throughout the day I was challenged and constantly drilled for eight hours. I figured, what is the worst that can happen? I didn't get the job but I was learning so much from him. Dr. Adam's purpose was to test my skills and knowledge of a potential NP in his department. Which we both know by the end of the day, I was not going to get hired for.

After the interview with Dr. Adam, I felt stupid and blamed myself for not getting the job. Different things kept running through my head. Why was I not confident with my answers? I knew what the answers were, why didn't I say them? Why was I so nervous? I still do not understand why I was so intimidated and nervous at the time. I believe my confidence level hit rock bottom from being unprepared. I continuously beat myself up for not getting the ED-NP position that I wanted so badly and desperately.

I finally decided to stop moping around and reminded myself, *what's done is done.* I needed to take the lessons I learned and apply them to my future interviews. I believe this bad interview lead me to great interviews in the future. While it was humiliating at the time, I learned many lessons about being prepared for future interviews.

Making your way to the interview

Before going to the interview, you will know how much the company will offer. The recruiter of the company will tell you the hourly rate or salary for the position. Remember, it is negotiable after you get the offer. Salary is mentioned in the forefront to avoid wasting each other's time.

I was contacted by a recruiter for an urgent care position. The recruiter went over my resume and thought that I would be a great fit for the company. After going through the introduction and asking me a few questions, she asked about my salary expectations. I told her "around the nineties annually but it is negotiable". The recruiter proceeded to tell me that they're around 70-80s and asked me if I was still interested. I told her that is about my salary as an RN currently. We thanked each other and hung up. Knowing that I wouldn't be making more than I was as an RN made me lose interest in the job and the recruiter wasn't willing to negotiate a higher wage.

Before beginning the job search, you also need to know what the average salary is in your area. A great website I checked for salary trends is http://www1.salary.com. You can narrow down your search to specialty and city.

Treat each interview like an important test and prepare for it.

I have learned a lot through my experience with Dr. Adam. I was not mentally prepared. I walked into the practice thinking, *I already have the job* and was overly confident. It is a good idea to get at least eight hours of sleep and eat a hardy meal before the interview. Looking back, I wasn't incompetent and didn't know my material, I was not mentally prepared. It is important to treat the interview or job shadow like taking a really important test. You have to give yourself a few days to prepare, write down questions, research the company, and go over any clinical information employers may ask. If you are interviewing for an infectious disease NP position, make sure you go over the infectious disease chapters and refresh your memory. Read a few recent articles and publications about infectious disease. I find that to be a great way to impress the employer and create a common ground to open up a line of communication.

Keep in mind each interview will be different from the last. The interview I had with a retail clinic and another ED practice, I was given a tour and a chance to ask questions then given the job. Another interview was with a mental health group. We met at Starbucks and it was very informal. Two weeks later, I was offered the mental health job. My personal philosophy is to be overly prepared and feel accomplish rather than underestimate the situation and look silly.

Ask questions during the interview.

The employer will always ask you if you have any questions. I highly recommend that you have at least five questions for the potential employer during the interview. Bring a list of questions, as this shows that you are interested in the position and prepared. I wrote down at least ten questions. You can use the same questions for multiple interviews, so don't be overwhelmed by the thought of having to think about new questions all the time.

Here are some examples of interview questions I have used in the past:

- How long is orientation for a new graduate NP?
- What are your requirements of full time nurse practitioner? What are your hours of operation? How many days per week is the practice open? Do you close for holidays? Do you have staff on call?
- How many providers are part of the practice? How many NPs or PAs?
- Are there career advancement opportunities available for a NP?
- Do you offer an allowance for continued medical education yearly?
- What are your expectations of me at three months, six months, and at one year?
- How will I be evaluated? Will you give me feedback along the way?
- Is there a bonus or increase in pay according to matrix such as patient's satisfaction score or number of patients being seen per hour?
- Is the practice affiliated with a teaching facility?
- Are there specialists or generalists available in the community for referral?

Being prepared with questions is a great way to show the interviewer that you have really thought about the job and what it requires. Showing interest in the company and the job will help you stand above other candidates. Think about great questions that pertain to the practice's specialty areas or possible patient base.

While the resume introduces your skills to a potential employer, the interview presents you as a person to them. You want to look professional, capable and knowledgeable. Being prepared for the interview and not going in with an inflated ego or high expectations will help you to be a more competitive candidate. Even if you don't get a job offer, take each experience as a learning one to use for the next interview!

Chapter 5- Seal the Deal

Depending on the company, you may be offered the job on the spot or there may be a waiting period where the employer will interview other candidates. When an on the spot job offer happens, you need to be prepared to either accept or decline the offer based upon what you know about the job. The skills I have obtained during the job search and interview process have helped me land a *same day* job offer of $130,000 a year! Finding the right job and the right interview techniques can make this happen for you as well! In this chapter, we are going to look at ways in which you can obtain job offers in the six digits right out of school!

Gather a portfolio

Like I mentioned earlier, you typically are aware of the salary before the interview with the hiring manager. I was contacted about an ER-NP position that pays $75 per hour with a commitment of only 144 hours a month. I was in disbelief when I heard this. I had to pull out my calculator to find out that is about $130,000 a year. I was thrilled! I had to ask the recruiter to repeat herself to make sure I heard it right. The average ER-NP rate in Atlanta, GA is about $50/hr. The job included a holiday bonus which is $112.5 an hour, a yearly stipend for continued education, overtime hours once I fulfilled my commitment, and a bonus depending on years of experience. The recruiter also warned me that the medical director, the person that makes the hiring decision, does not typically hire new graduates. However, the medical director liked my resume and wanted to meet me.

I scheduled the interview for a week later. I wanted to be prepared for anything. I treated this interview like I was taking my national NP boards all over again. I reviewed the most common ER case studies. I read emergency medicine physician journals. I did extensive research about the company. I did everything I mentioned in this book. The one thing I did differently on this interview was I created a portfolio. I believe the portfolio led to the same day offer.

My portfolio consisted of my resume, recommendation letters, and a case and procedural log. You can put anything in the portfolio, but I like to keep mine short, sweet and "to-the-point". I feel medical directors do not have much time, and I just want to give them the facts. I had two letters of recommendation. One was from an ER physician whom I worked with and observed me while I was in school. The second letter was from an ER-NP whom I worked with and who guided me through my NP education. I had known both of them for over three years and had had good working relationship with them. I strongly suggest you bring a few recommendation letters with you on the interview if possible. The recommendation letters will set you apart from other candidates and serve as expert testimonies regarding your ability to perform and excel at the job.

I also printed out my case log and procedural log that I was obligated to keep while going through my NP track. My school used software called Typhon Group Healthcare Solutions. I know most NP programs use Typhon or something similar. The software allowed me to print out a .pdf of all the patients logged and the procedures that I did while in clinical. This is a great tool to show your potential employer. This is concrete evidence of your qualifications and skills. The recommendation letters and case log are great resources to increase the chances of getting hired.

I met with the medical director. We started talking and she asked me some general questions such as tell me about yourself and why do I want to be an ER-NP. Then she proceeded to asking me clinical questions and case scenarios. I was mentally ready and did well. *Thanks to Dr. Adam,* I thought. She then proceeded to see if I had any questions. I asked her at least five of the questions that I mentioned earlier in the book. I also asked a few questions about the company and stated some facts I had read about the company on their website. The medical director seemed impressed. Toward the end of the interview, I handed her my portfolio. I told her it has my recommendation letters and my case log during my NP training. She smiled and was very impressed.

She got the recruiter to give me a tour of the department. The staff all seemed very friendly. While touring with the recruiter, I asked about the RN and provider turnover rate. I assessed the working environment and case load of the RNs. There were three NPs and two PAs working in the department. One of the PAs was moving and this left one vacancy. Most of the advanced practice providers, who were either PA or NP, had been with the company for over five years. I got the opportunity to speak with the PA who was leaving. I asked about her job satisfaction and challenges within the department. I got great feedback from her. At that moment, I knew I wanted to work here. When the recruiter and I rounded back to the front, the medical director was at the front and she offered me the job. At that moment, I thought it was so unreal. I have never been to an interview and received an offer the same day! It was pure bliss!

This can happen to you too. You have to make yourself marketable. There are a lot of good NP jobs available but they can be very difficult to get due to there being so many applicants. You have to make yourself stand out. Get creative. Show them that you want the job and are willing to go the extra mile to get it. By doing so, you are also showing that you are willing to go the extra mile for your patients.

Chapter 6- Keep Your Options Open

While you might not get a same day offer such as the one that I received, there are still great opportunities out there for you. You just have to find them. Keeping your options open and being flexible will boost your chances at finding a good NP job. Be open to new ideas and what you're willing to do to get the job you want.

If the market for NP in your area is too competitive, is commuting an option?

I live in a busy downtown area in Atlanta, Georgia. The job market in Atlanta is extremely competitive, with a flood of nurse practitioners coming out of school. I found it difficult to get a job or get the salary I wanted in my local area. The average salary for an NP in Georgia is about $87k. My salary goal was at least $90k. I received some offers around Atlanta for less than what I was making as an RN. I received an offer at an urgent care practice for $34 per hour from 5pm to 11pm Monday- Friday without benefits. I thought to myself, *I'm making more as an RN right now.* Therefore, I decided to look further away from the city. Instead of a 60 mile radius, I put down 100 mile radius in the search engines. I am in Atlanta, where traffic is always something to consider. If I am willing to travel 100 miles, I pick areas that are against the traffic. You might be surprised that the further you are from the city, the salary may increase. In my case, it did. All because I was flexible with my search criteria.

Negotiate your contract

Once you have the offer—negotiate! When talking to other providers, most people seem to accept the offer that is originally given to them. Bad mistake. Always negotiate. With one company, I negotiated from $50/hr to $60/hr because I chose to opt out of healthcare benefits. Now, some companies do not give you the option to opt-out, but you don't know until you ask. I did not take the job, but knowing that they were flexible with terms of the contract helped me find ways that I could negotiate my future contracts to fit my needs.

I know two other NPs who are new graduates and both work for the same company. Both hold the same degree and perform the same tasks with the same level of experience. One person negotiated her contract and her base pay to $90k annually. Whereas, the other person accepted the offer at $85k annually. Now, I am not telling you to overdo it. I believe negotiating around $5k is reasonable. However, some companies have a set mark for years of experience and that is non-negotiable. For example, a retail clinic offered me $45/hr. When I tried to negotiate, the recruiter told me they start all new NP graduates the same and it is corporate policies. I understood and moved on. It is always good to ask. The worst case scenario is that they say "no." It is very unlikely they will retract the offer of employment if you are trying to negotiate pay.

Knowing what you are willing to do and where you are willing to look can open up even greater possibilities for your job offers. Take the time to figure out how far you are willing to go and try to negotiate the terms of the offered contract so that you can get the best terms possible. The right job is out there for you. Don't be discouraged if it doesn't show itself right away.

Chapter 7- A Word Based Upon My Experience

During your job search or after passing the national boards, it is a good idea to apply for a state license as an NP. Each state may be different in its requirements, but in Georgia, it typically takes about three to four weeks to get state certified. Visit your state board of nursing website for more information about certification.

You can also apply for a National Provider Identifier (NPI) number. An NPI is a unique 10-digit number issued to health care providers by the Centers for Medicare and Medicaid Services (CMS) for billing. Look at the link below and create an account. It typically takes less than a week to get your NPI number.

https://nppes.cms.hhs.gov/NPPES/Welcome.do

Depending on the state, you can not apply for a DEA number without meeting certain protocol and having a sponsoring physician. I work in Georgia and cannot apply for it until I have a sponsoring physician. Also, if you wait for the job offer, some employers will pay for your DEA number, which is about $700. I would wait until you get the job and meet all the criteria. Also, some employers, such as retail clinics, do not require a DEA number, so you do not need one.

Knowledge is power. Know what you need to do for your state and your area before just going forward with licenses and certifications. Some of these can be costly and unnecessary for you to succeed in your job. You negotiated a great salary, don't waste it on things that you really don't need.

Conclusion

I have been in my new job for a few months now and absolutely love it. The pay is nice, but I also love knowing that I am making a difference in someone else's life. When I made my decision to become an NP, I wanted to be able to do more for my patients than I could as an RN. Now that I have the job, I have found that I am much more fulfilled than I was as an RN.

Yes, working and raising two young children is difficult, but I know what my hours are and have a routine now. I constantly keep my portfolio and resume updated just in case something better should arise.

I hope this book has been an encouragement to you in your journey to becoming a NP. With such a competitive field before you, you want to have all the tools you can get in order to make sure you stand the best chance at getting the best job possible.

Good luck in your job search!

www.ingramcontent.com/pod-product-compliance
Lightning Source LLC
Chambersburg PA
CBHW041614180526
45159CB00002BC/850